THE COMPLETE ESOPHAGITIS DIET COOKBOOK FOR BEGINNERS

Eat Your Way to Symptom Relief, Improved Digestion, Eliminating Acid Reflux, Losing Weight, and Preventing Complications

Daria Cross, RD

COPYRIGHT PAGE

The information in this book is not intended, under any circumstances, to replace or serve as a substitute for professional medical advice, diagnosis, or treatment. Any individual seeking advice regarding a medical condition or seeking treatment options should always consult with a qualified healthcare provider or physician. The author and publisher explicitly disclaim any responsibility for adverse effects or consequences arising from the utilization of the recipes or information presented in this cookbook.

Table of Contents

Introduction to Esophagitis

Esophagitis is an inflammation or irritation of the esophagus, the tube that carries food from your mouth to your stomach. This condition can cause symptoms such as pain while swallowing, heartburn, and a sensation of something being stuck in your throat. It may feel sore, swollen, raw, or burning. Esophagitis results from the immune system's response to infections, allergens, or tissue damage, and can also be caused by erosive substances like stomach acid and certain medications.

There are several types of esophagitis, each with its own specific causes and symptoms. Common causes include acid reflux, infections, certain medications, and allergens. If left untreated, esophagitis can lead to complications such as painful swallowing, chest pain, nausea, bleeding, aspiration pneumonia, or strictures and tears in the esophagus.

Treatment for esophagitis typically involves addressing the underlying cause of the inflammation and avoiding triggers like specific foods or allergens. Medications, dietary changes, and sometimes surgery may be necessary to manage the condition. With prompt diagnosis and appropriate treatment, the outlook for esophagitis is generally positive.

PART 1: OVERVIEW OF THE ESOPHAGUS

Esophagitis refers to inflammation or injury to the lining of the esophagus, the tube connecting the throat to the stomach. One of the primary culprits behind this condition is gastroesophageal reflux, commonly known as acid reflux, which can lead to erosive esophagitis. Other causes include radiation, infections, medication-induced local injury (such as pill esophagitis), and eosinophilic esophagitis (EoE). Symptoms of esophagitis typically include chest pain, painful swallowing (odynophagia), and difficulty swallowing (dysphagia). Patients with EoE may experience food impaction. In severe cases, esophagitis can result in complications such as strictures, fistulas, or perforation, each presenting with its own set of symptoms.

Reflux esophagitis, where stomach acids flow back up into the esophagus due to a malfunctioning lower esophageal sphincter, is a common cause. This sphincter is a ring of muscle located at the lower end of the esophagus, responsible for preventing stomach contents from refluxing upwards. Factors contributing to reflux esophagitis may include the presence of a hiatal hernia, where part of the stomach protrudes into the chest cavity. Certain foods with high acidic content, like red salsa, onions, alcohol, and citrus fruits or juices, can exacerbate symptoms.

Untreated esophagitis can have serious implications, potentially progressing to Barrett's esophagus, a condition linked to an increased risk of esophageal cancer. Management of esophagitis varies depending on the underlying cause and may involve prescription medications, dietary adjustments, or even surgical intervention.

Living with esophagitis not only brings physical discomfort but can also take a toll on emotional well-being. Individuals diagnosed with certain types of esophagitis may be at a heightened risk of experiencing anxiety and depression. Thus, prompt diagnosis and management are essential not only for symptom relief but also for overall health and quality of life.

Importance of Early Diagnosis and Treatment

Recognizing and treating esophagitis early on is really important for managing this condition effectively and avoiding potential complications. Esophagitis, which is basically inflammation or injury to the lining of the esophagus, can cause a lot of discomfort with symptoms like chest pain and trouble swallowing.

One big reason we want to catch it early is so we can figure out what's causing it and deal with that right away. Whether it's because of acid reflux, certain medications, infections, or something else, knowing the root cause helps us choose the best treatment. For example, if it's caused by acid reflux, we can work on managing that to ease symptoms and stop more damage to the esophagus.

Getting in there early also lowers the chances of things getting worse. Left untreated, esophagitis can lead to more serious problems like narrowing of the esophagus, holes, or even tears. But by tackling the inflammation early, we can lower the risk of these complications and make life a lot easier for folks dealing with this condition.

Plus, starting treatment sooner means we can help people feel better faster. Dealing with symptoms like chest pain and heartburn can be a real pain, so getting them under control early on can make a big difference in how someone feels day to day.

And let's not forget about the long-term benefits. By nipping esophagitis in the bud, we can also lower the chances of it turning into something more serious, like Barrett's esophagus, which increases the risk of esophageal cancer. So, catching and treating esophagitis early isn't just about feeling better now—it's about staying healthier in the long run.

Types of Esophagitis

Esophagitis comes in various forms, each with its own set of causes and characteristics:

1. Erosive or Reflux Esophagitis:

This is one of the most common types, where stomach contents flow back into the esophagus due to a faulty valve. Known as gastroesophageal reflux disease (GERD), this backflow can damage the esophageal lining, especially if it occurs frequently.

2. Eosinophilic or Autoimmune Esophagitis:

Often associated with allergies, this type occurs when too many eosinophils, a type of white blood cell, accumulate in the esophageal lining. Certain foods like milk, eggs, soy, and wheat may trigger this condition.

3. Lymphocytic Esophagitis:

Characterized by an excess of lymphocytes (another type of white blood cell) in the esophagus, this condition may be related to eosinophilic esophagitis or GERD.

4. Drug-induced Esophagitis:

Certain medications, when not properly swallowed or in contact with the esophageal tissue for an extended period, can cause damage. Pain relievers like aspirin and ibuprofen, antibiotics, and drugs used for heart problems or osteoporosis are among the culprits.

5. Infectious Esophagitis:

Caused by viruses, bacteria, or fungi, this type of esophagitis is more common in individuals with weakened immune systems, such as those with cancer or HIV/AIDS. Candida albicans, a fungus found in the mouth, is a common cause, especially in individuals taking steroids or antibiotics or those with diabetes.

6. Radiation Esophagitis:

Resulting from radiation therapy for cancer, this type of esophagitis can damage the esophageal tissue.

Understanding the specific type of esophagitis is crucial for determining the appropriate treatment approach and managing symptoms effectively. Whether it's addressing underlying conditions, avoiding trigger foods, or using medication, early recognition and intervention can significantly improve outcomes for individuals with esophagitis.

Causes and Risk Factors

The lining of the esophagus is quite sensitive, making it prone to irritation and inflammation. Your esophagus tissues might become inflamed if your immune system has been activated to fight an infection, if you're having an allergic reaction or if something corrosive has injured the tissues.

Various factors can heighten the risk of developing esophagitis:

Refluxed Stomach Acid: Individuals with gastroesophageal reflux disease (GERD) may experience leakage of stomach acid into the esophagus due to a malfunctioning muscle at the esophageal end. This reflux can be triggered by factors like pregnancy, obesity, smoking, alcohol consumption, carbonated beverages, or consumption of fatty or spicy foods.

Excessive Vomiting: Acid present in vomit can irritate the esophagus, leading to inflammation. Persistent or excessive vomiting can exacerbate this condition.

Medication Use: Certain medications, such as aspirin, nonsteroidal anti-inflammatory drugs (NSAIDs) like ibuprofen and naproxen, antibiotics, vitamin C supplements, and potassium chloride, can damage the esophageal lining if they remain in contact with it for extended periods. This can occur when pills are not properly swallowed with enough water.

Infections: Viral infections like herpes simplex virus, yeast (Candida), or bacterial infections can cause esophageal irritation. This is more common in individuals with weakened immune systems, such as those with HIV/AIDS or recent organ transplants, but can also occur in individuals with normal immune function.

Chemical Irritation: Accidental or intentional ingestion of strong chemicals, such as household bleach, drain cleaner, or detergent, can injure the esophagus. The severity of the irritation increases with prolonged exposure to the chemical.

Radiation Injury: Radiation therapy for cancer, particularly in the chest or neck region, can lead to esophagitis as the sensitive lining of the esophagus becomes inflamed or thins out due to radiation exposure.

Systemic Illnesses: Certain systemic conditions like scleroderma, inflammatory bowel disease (IBD), Behçet's disease, or Sjögren's syndrome can contribute to the development of esophagitis.

Allergic/Immune Response: Esophageal reactions to foods or irritants can contribute to the development of eosinophilic esophagitis, a chronic autoimmune disease.

Understanding these contributing factors is crucial for effectively managing esophagitis and minimizing its impact on overall health and well-being.

PART 2: SYMPTOMS OF ESOPHAGITIS

Experiencing esophagitis often brings about common symptoms like heartburn, difficulty swallowing, or pain during swallowing. Other indicators may include:

- A sore throat

- Sensation of something stuck in the throat

- Burning feeling in the esophagus

- Coughing

- Hoarseness

- Nausea or vomiting

- Fever

The intensity of pain can vary from mild to severe and may be intermittent or persistent. Depending on the cause and severity, you might also notice:

- Acid reflux

- Regurgitation

- Difficulty swallowing food

- Indigestion

- Feeding difficulties, particularly in children

- Presence of blood in vomit

- Mouth sores

In babies and children, symptoms may include:

- Feeding difficulties, such as refusing to eat, showing irritability, or arching their back during feeding

- Failure to gain weight

- Chest or abdominal pain in older children

Advanced stages of esophagitis may involve bleeding in the esophagus.

Complications of Esophagitis

When left untreated, esophagitis can lead to significant health complications affecting the function and structure of the esophagus. Some of these complications include:

- Esophageal strictures, where the esophagus narrows, making it difficult to swallow.

- Esophageal perforation, a rare but serious condition where there's a hole or tear in the esophagus.

- Laryngitis, characterized by inflammation of the vocal cords, leading to hoarseness or loss of voice.

- Aspiration pneumonia, a lung infection resulting from inhaling food, stomach acid, or saliva into the lungs.

- Scarring or narrowing of the esophagus, known as a stricture, which can further impair swallowing.

- Tearing of the esophageal lining due to retching or passage of instruments during endoscopy, potentially leading to bleeding or infection.

- Barrett's esophagus, a condition where the cells lining the esophagus are damaged by acid reflux, increasing the risk of esophageal cancer.

These complications underscore the importance of timely diagnosis and treatment of esophagitis to prevent long-term consequences and improve overall health outcomes.

Diagnosis of Esophagitis

Your healthcare provider or specialist will typically diagnose esophagitis by conducting a thorough assessment, which may include:

Endoscopy:

During this procedure, a slender tube with a tiny camera, known as an endoscope, is gently guided down your throat and into the esophagus. Your provider examines the esophagus for any abnormalities and may take small tissue samples, called biopsies, for further analysis. You'll receive light sedation to ensure comfort during the test.

Esophageal Sponge Test:

This test can be conducted in the healthcare provider's office. It involves swallowing a capsule attached to a string. After dissolving in your stomach, the capsule releases a sponge that your provider retrieves through your mouth using the string. The sponge collects samples of esophageal tissue, aiding in assessing inflammation levels without the need for an endoscopy.

Barium X-ray:

In this procedure, you'll drink a solution or ingest a pill containing barium, a contrast material. Barium coats the esophageal and stomach lining, allowing for clear imaging of these organs. This helps identify structural changes, narrowing of the esophagus, hiatal hernias, tumors, or other irregularities contributing to symptoms.

Allergy Testing:

If allergic or immune reactions are suspected as the cause of esophagitis, your provider may conduct allergy tests such as skin prick tests, blood tests, or food patch testing. These tests help pinpoint specific food or environmental allergens triggering the condition.

Laboratory Tests:

Tissue samples obtained during endoscopy are sent to the lab for analysis. Depending on the suspected cause, laboratory tests may be performed to diagnose bacterial, viral, or fungal infections, as well as identify irregular cells indicating esophageal cancer or precancerous changes.

Treatment Options

Treatment for esophagitis aims to alleviate symptoms, manage complications, and address underlying causes. Treatment approaches vary depending on the cause of the condition.

For reflux esophagitis, treatment may involve:

- Nonprescription treatments like antacids, H-2-receptor blockers (e.g., cimetidine), and proton pump inhibitors (e.g., lansoprazole, omeprazole).

- Prescription medicines, including stronger H-2-receptor blockers and proton pump inhibitors.

- Surgical options like fundoplication or the LINX procedure, which involves placing a ring of magnetic beads around the lower esophageal sphincter to prevent acid reflux.

For eosinophilic esophagitis, treatment typically includes:

- Proton pump inhibitors to reduce acid production.

- Steroids such as fluticasone or budesonide, which can be swallowed to target esophageal tissue inflammation.

- Elimination or elemental diets to identify and avoid trigger foods.

- Monoclonal antibodies like dupilumab, which block proteins causing inflammation and are administered via injection.

For drug-induced esophagitis, treatment involves:

- Avoiding the problematic drug whenever possible.

- Using alternative medications that are less likely to cause esophagitis.

- Taking medications in liquid form if available.

- Ensuring proper pill-taking habits, including swallowing pills with a full glass of water and remaining upright for at least 30 minutes after ingestion.

In cases of infectious esophagitis, treatment may include:

- Prescription medications to target bacterial, viral, fungal, or parasitic infections.

For common complications like esophageal narrowing, a gastroenterologist may perform esophageal dilation using endoscopic devices.

These devices may feature a tapered tip or an expandable balloon to widen the esophagus when severe narrowing or food impaction occurs.

Overall, treatment strategies are tailored to individual needs and may involve a combination of medication, dietary adjustments, lifestyle modifications, and medical procedures to effectively manage esophagitis and its complications.

Long-term Management Strategies

Lifestyle Adjustments:

Maintain a healthy weight to ease pressure on your stomach and esophagus.

Elevate the head of your bed to prevent nighttime heartburn.

Avoid lying down or bending over after meals.

Opt for smaller, more frequent meals to reduce stomach pressure.

Identify and steer clear of trigger foods like spicy dishes, citrus fruits, caffeine, alcohol, and fizzy drinks.

Quit smoking to protect your lower esophageal sphincter from weakening.

Dietary Changes:

Stick to a diet low in acid and fat to soothe your esophagus.

Boost your fiber intake to prevent constipation, a common reflux trigger.

Stay hydrated by drinking plenty of water throughout the day.

Medication Management:

Take prescribed medications exactly as directed by your doctor, whether it's proton pump inhibitors (PPIs), H-2 receptor blockers, or antacids, to manage stomach acid and alleviate symptoms.

If you're dealing with eosinophilic esophagitis, stick to your treatment plan, which might involve proton pump inhibitors, swallowed steroids, or eliminating trigger foods.

Regular Check-Ins:

Keep up with your scheduled check-ups with your healthcare provider to monitor your condition and fine-tune your treatment regimen.

Don't hesitate to reach out if you notice any new or worsening symptoms.

Stress Management:

Incorporate stress-relieving techniques into your routine, like relaxation exercises, mindfulness, yoga, or deep breathing, to help keep stress-induced symptoms at bay.

Avoiding Irritants:

Steer clear of environmental irritants such as air pollution or harsh chemicals, which can inflame your esophagus.

Endoscopic Surveillance:

If you're at risk for esophageal cancer due to conditions like Barrett's esophagus, your doctor may recommend regular endoscopic check-ups to monitor any changes in your esophageal lining.

Seek Support:

Don't hesitate to lean on healthcare professionals, support groups, or online communities for guidance and emotional support as you navigate life with esophagitis.

By integrating these strategies into your daily routine and staying in tune with your body's needs, you can effectively manage esophagitis and enjoy a better quality of life in the long run.

PART 3: ESOPHAGITIS AND DIET

Esophagitis can often heal on its own, but adopting an esophageal or soft food diet can help ease discomfort and speed up recovery. Here are some tips for following a soft diet:

- Take small, well-chewed bites of food to make swallowing easier.

- Avoid tough meats, hard bread, and abrasive foods that can irritate the esophagus.

- Sip fluids with meals to moisten food and aid in swallowing.

- Stop eating when you feel full to prevent overfilling the stomach.

- Eat slowly in a relaxed setting to aid digestion.

- Opt for decaffeinated beverages and avoid very hot or cold drinks.

- Sit upright while eating and remain seated for 45-60 minutes after meals.

- Avoid eating for at least 3 hours before bedtime.

- Eat smaller, more frequent meals and snacks throughout the day.

When planning your soft food diet, focus on easily digestible foods and steer clear of carbonated drinks. Your healthcare provider may recommend limiting citrus, mint, or caffeinated beverages. Here are some dietary suggestions:

Dairy:

- Choose softer cheeses like cream cheese, brie, Neufchâtel, and ricotta.

- Opt for plain yogurt without added fruit, granola, or seeds.

- Low-fat ice cream can be enjoyed if cold foods don't aggravate symptoms.

Fiber:

- Replace raw fruits and vegetables with canned or frozen options like applesauce, fruit cups, avocados, and bananas.

- Include soups and broths to soften vegetables like squash, potatoes, and carrots, avoiding fibrous or seeded varieties.

Breads and Grains:

- Soften bread and crackers in soups or broths.

- Opt for cooked cereals without nuts or seeds.

- Avoid hard bread crusts, muffins, dinner rolls, and rice.

Proteins:

- Choose ground or pureed beef, pork, and poultry to protect the esophagus.

- Enjoy boneless white fish like cod and tilapia.

- Consider soft scrambled eggs or egg substitutes.

If esophagitis is a symptom of an underlying condition, maintaining good nutrition is essential for overall health. Consult your healthcare provider for personalized dietary recommendations and guidelines tailored to your specific needs.

Objectives of an Esophagitis-Friendly Diet

1. **Soothe Irritation and Inflammation:** When dealing with esophagitis, the focus is on calming down the inflammation and irritation in the esophagus. This means steering clear of foods and

drinks known to trigger inflammation, like acidic fruits, spicy dishes, and fatty foods.

2. **Make Swallowing Easier:** Esophagitis can make swallowing a real challenge due to the inflammation and narrowing of the esophagus. To help with this, the diet leans towards softer, easier-to-chew foods that slide down smoothly. The aim is to prevent any food from getting stuck along the way.

3. **Avoid Food Blockages:** There's nothing worse than feeling like your food is stuck in your throat. That's why the diet focuses on foods less likely to cause blockages, such as well-cooked veggies, tender meats, and softer grains. This helps ensure everything goes down without a hitch.

4. **Ease Those Symptoms:** Heartburn, chest pain, and trouble swallowing are all too common with

esophagitis. By avoiding foods and drinks that trigger acid reflux and including soothing options, like herbal teas and gentle soups, the diet aims to ease these uncomfortable symptoms.

5. **Support Healing and Recovery:** To help the esophagus heal up, the diet is packed with foods rich in vitamins, minerals, and antioxidants. These nutrients are essential for repairing tissues and boosting the immune system, so you can bounce back from esophagitis stronger than ever.

By sticking to these guidelines, an Esophagitis-Friendly Diet can help manage symptoms, reduce the risk of complications, and support your overall health as you recover from esophagitis.

Foods to Avoid

High-fat meals often slow down digestion, which can exacerbate symptoms of GERD. Additionally, highly acidic foods can increase stomach acid, further irritating the esophagus. A GERD-friendly diet aims to avoid foods that are likely to trigger reflux and worsen symptoms.

Citrus fruits like oranges, grapefruits, and sometimes pineapples are common reflux triggers due to their high acid content.

The high acidity of tomatoes and tomato-based foods can be irritating to the esophagus, so it's best to avoid them.

Whole milk, cream, ice cream, and full-fat yogurt can increase stomach acid and relax the esophageal sphincter, leading to reflux.

High-fat and heavily processed meats such as bacon, sausages, hot dogs, hamburgers, salami, pastrami, and pepperoni should be avoided. Similarly, steer clear of fried or greasy foods like French fries and fried chicken, as well as rich sauces or gravies.

Mint, especially peppermint, can cause discomfort by relaxing the esophageal sphincter and increasing reflux.

Chocolate can increase stomach acid, so it's best to avoid candies, desserts, or baked goods containing it, including hot chocolate.

Spices such as cinnamon, curry powder, chili powder, cayenne pepper, and hot paprika can be irritating. Cuisines heavily seasoned with these spices, like Mexican, Thai, and Indian, should be avoided.

Carbonated beverages can be bothersome, regardless of caffeine content. Coffee and alcohol both increase stomach acid and can irritate the stomach and esophagus, so they should be avoided.

Recommended Foods and Nutrients

Most fruits are good choices, except for citrus fruits which are known to trigger symptoms in some individuals. Berries, melons, apples, pears, and bananas are generally safe options unless you notice specific sensitivities.

Vegetables are excellent for increasing fiber intake, which is beneficial for digestion. However, avoid tomatoes, tomato sauce, and spicy peppers as they can be irritating. Some people also find onions and garlic aggravating, so pay attention to your body's reactions.

Incorporate a variety of whole grains like oats, brown rice, quinoa, farro, 100% whole wheat, and wheat bran into your diet. These grains are rich in fiber and can help with digestion. Aim to include a small serving with each meal.

Opt for low-fat or non-fat dairy options, or choose non-dairy alternatives like almond milk, soy milk, or coconut milk. These are less likely to trigger GERD symptoms compared to full-fat dairy products.

Choose lean cuts of beef or pork, skinless poultry, and seafood. These proteins are less likely to cause reflux compared to higher-fat meats.

Incorporate healthy fats such as olive oil, avocados, nuts, nut butters, and seeds like pumpkin and chia into your diet. These fats are beneficial when consumed in moderation and can help reduce inflammation.

Stick to fresh or dried herbs like basil, parsley, oregano, and thyme. These add flavor without the risk of triggering reflux that comes with stronger spices.

Soy products like edamame, tofu, tempeh, miso, and soy nuts are great meat alternatives. They are generally lower in fat and free of cholesterol, making them suitable for a GERD diet.

Beans, peas, lentils, chickpeas, and other legumes are excellent sources of protein and fiber. They can be added to various recipes to enhance both nutrition and flavor.

Stay hydrated with plain or fruit-infused water. Caffeine-free herbal teas containing ginger, licorice, or fennel can soothe your digestive system.

In a study published in the World Journal of Gastroenterology, individuals with heartburn who incorporated 15 grams of psyllium fiber supplements daily experienced increased esophageal sphincter pressure, fewer acid reflux incidents, and reduced heartburn symptoms.

To boost your fiber intake, aim to fill half of your plate with an assortment of GERD-friendly fruits and vegetables during meals and snacks. This not only helps manage symptoms but also promotes overall digestive health.

Post-Meal Practices

After a meal, it's crucial for individuals dealing with esophagitis to follow practices that aid in comfort and reduce the risk of worsening symptoms. Here are some helpful post-meal habits:

1. **Stay Upright:** Avoid lying down immediately after eating. Instead, remain upright or engage in light activities like walking to encourage proper digestion and minimize the chance of acid reflux.

2. **Avoid Tight Clothing**: Opt for loose-fitting clothing, especially around the waist, to prevent putting pressure on the stomach and exacerbating acid reflux.

3. **Stay Hydrated:** Drink non-acidic beverages like water to help wash down food and prevent throat dryness. Steer clear of carbonated or caffeinated drinks, as they can worsen symptoms.

4. **Chew Thoroughly:** Take your time to chew food thoroughly before swallowing to aid in digestion and prevent irritation to the esophagus.

5. **Steer Clear of Trigger Foods**: Identify and avoid foods known to trigger esophagitis symptoms, such

as spicy, acidic, or caffeinated items, as well as chocolate and alcohol. Opt for gentler, non-irritating options whenever possible.

6. **Gentle Movement:** Engage in light physical activities like walking or gentle stretching after eating to aid digestion. Avoid intense exercise immediately after meals, as it may worsen symptoms.

7. **Consider Medication Timing:** Follow your healthcare provider's instructions on when to take medication for esophagitis in relation to meals, as some medications work better when taken before or after eating.

8. **Monitor Symptoms**: Pay attention to how you feel after eating and note any triggers or patterns in your symptoms. This information can help you make informed decisions about diet and lifestyle adjustments.

9. **Manage Stress:** Incorporate relaxation techniques such as deep breathing or meditation into your post-meal routine to reduce stress, which can exacerbate esophagitis symptoms.

10. **Elevate Your Upper Body:** If nighttime reflux is a concern, consider elevating the head of your bed or using extra pillows to keep your upper body raised while sleeping. This helps prevent stomach acid from flowing back into the esophagus while lying down.

By following these post-meal practices, individuals with esophagitis can alleviate discomfort and promote better digestive health. Always consult with a healthcare provider for personalized advice and treatment options.

PART 4: TASTY RECIPES FOR ESOPHAGITIS-FRIENDLY MEALS

ESOPHAGITIS-FRIENDLY BREAKFAST RECIPES

Chai tea

<u>Ingredients</u>

2 mugs milk (or use almond milk)

2 English Breakfast tea bags

6 cracked cardamom pods

½ cinnamon stick

a grating of fresh nutmeg

2 cloves

2-4 tsp light brown soft sugar

How to Make

STEP 1

Heat the milk in a saucepan over a very low heat. Empty the contents of the tea bags into the pan, then add the cracked cardamom pods, cinnamon stick, nutmeg and cloves.

STEP 2

Sweeten with light brown soft sugar to taste (chai tea should be sweet, but use less if you like), then leave to infuse, but not boil, for 10 mins. Strain into mugs and enjoy.

Cinnamon cashew flapjacks

Ingredients

140g butter, plus extra for greasing

140g light brown soft sugar

2 tbsp set honey

1 tbsp ground cinnamon

140g porridge oats

85g desiccated coconut

85g sesame seeds

50g sunflower seeds

1 tbsp plain flour

85g cashews or pecans

How to Make

STEP 1

Heat oven to 160C/140C fan/gas 3. Grease and line a 20 x 30cm cake tin with baking parchment. Melt the butter in a large non-stick pan, add the sugar, honey and cinnamon, and stir with a wooden spoon over a low heat for 5-10 mins until the sugar dissolves.

STEP 2

Remove from the heat and stir in all the remaining **Ingredients** until well coated in the buttery spice mixture. Tip into the tin and press down to an even layer. Bake for 30-35 mins until golden. Cool for 5 mins, then mark into squares – don't remove from the tin yet as they won't hold together until they are cold. Will keep in a sealed container for a couple of days.

Creamy mushrooms on toast

<u>**Ingredients**</u>

1 slice wholemeal bread

1 ½ tbsp light cream cheese

1 tsp rapeseed oil

3handfuls sliced, small flat mushrooms

2 tbsp skimmed milk

¼ tsp wholegrain mustard

1 tbsp snipped chives

How to Make

STEP 1

Toast the bread, then spread with a little of the cream cheese.

STEP 2

Meanwhile, heat the oil in a non-stick pan and cook the mushrooms, stirring frequently, until softened. Spoon in the milk, remaining cheese and the mustard. Stir well until coated. Tip onto the toast and top with chives.

Winter breakfast hash

Ingredients

375g potatoes, cut into small chunks

1 tbsp rapeseed oil

1 onion (about 200g), chopped

½ tsp caraway seeds

2 garlic cloves, chopped

1 green pepper, deseeded and diced

200g large brussels sprouts, trimmed and sliced

2 eggs

<u>How to Make</u>

STEP 1

Boil the potatoes for 15 mins until tender. Meanwhile, heat the oil in a large non-stick frying pan over a medium heat and fry the onion for 8 mins, stirring frequently until it starts to colour. Add the caraway, garlic, pepper and sprouts and cook for 5 mins more with the lid on the pan so they steam at the same time.

STEP 2

Drain and lightly crush the cooked potatoes using a masher. Stir them into the vegetables and cook for 5-10 mins, turning occasionally so the mixture browns.

STEP 3

Meanwhile, poach the eggs for a few minutes for a runny yolk or until cooked to your liking. Remove from the pan using a slotted spoon. Serve each portion of hash topped with an egg.

Herb omelette with fried tomatoes

Ingredients

1 tsp olive oil

3 tomatoes, halved

4 large eggs

1 tbsp chopped parsley

1 tbsp chopped basil

How to Make

STEP 1

Heat the oil in a small non-stick frying pan, then cook the tomatoes cut-side down until starting to soften and colour. Meanwhile, beat the eggs with the herbs and plenty of freshly ground black pepper in a small bowl.

STEP 2

Scoop the tomatoes from the pan and put them on two serving plates. Pour the egg mixture into the pan and stir gently with a wooden spoon so the egg that sets on the base of the pan moves to enable uncooked egg to flow into the space. Stop stirring when it's nearly cooked to allow it to set into an omelette. Cut into four and serve with the tomatoes.

Baked eggs brunch

<u>Ingredients</u>

2 tbsp olive oil

2 leeks, thinly sliced

2 onions, thinly sliced

2 x 100g bags baby spinach leaves

handful fresh wholemeal breadcrumbs

25g parmesan (or vegetarian alternative), finely grated

4 sundried tomatoes, chopped

4 medium eggs

How to Make

STEP 1

Heat oven to 200C/180C fan/gas 6. Heat the oil in a pan and add the leeks, onions and seasoning. Cook for 15-20 mins until soft and beginning to caramelise.

STEP 2

Meanwhile, put the spinach in a colander and pour over a kettle of boiling water. When cool enough to handle, squeeze out as much liquid as possible. Mix the breadcrumbs and cheese together.

STEP 3

Arrange the leek and onion mixture between 4 ovenproof dishes, then scatter with the spinach and pieces of sundried tomato. Make a well in the middle of each dish and crack an egg in it. Season and sprinkle with cheese crumbs. Put the dishes on a baking tray and cook for 12-15 mins, until the whites are set and yolks are cooked to your liking.

Panettone French toast

<u>Ingredients</u>

3 eggs

150ml whole milk

1 tsp mixed spice

2 tbsp double cream

3 tbsp brandy

40g unsalted butter

4 tbsp mixed dried fruit

4 slices panettone (around 320g), cut in half to make 8

60g crème fraîche, to serve

maple syrup, to serve (optional)

2 tsp icing sugar, to serve

How to Make

STEP 1

Tip the eggs, milk, mixed spice, double cream and 1 tbsp brandy into a jug and beat to combine, then pour the mixture into a large, shallow dish.

STEP 2

Pour the remaining brandy into a cold frying pan along with 15g butter and the mixed fruit. Warm over a low heat for 3-4 mins until the butter has melted and the liquid has thickened slightly. Pour the fruit mixture into a small heatproof bowl and set aside.

STEP 3

Lay the panettone slices in the egg mixture and flip over to soak. Do this quickly so it doesn't break apart. Set aside on a plate.

STEP 4

Melt the remaining butter over a medium-low heat in the frying pan you used earlier, and fry the panettone slices for 3-4 mins on each side until golden and cooked through. It's easier to do this over a lower heat so the outside doesn't burn before the centre cooks.

STEP 5

Divide the slices between four plates, then top with the crème fraîche, mixed fruit, a little maple syrup (if using) and a dusting of icing sugar.

Fruity coconut creams

Ingredients

1 x 50g/2oz sachet coconut cream

500g 0% Greek yogurt or tub quark

85g icing sugar, sieved

few drops vanilla extract

2 kiwi fruit

400g can pineapple chunks

How to Make

STEP 1

Dissolve the coconut cream in 50ml boiling water, then leave to cool. Spoon the quark or yogurt into a mixing bowl, then stir in the icing sugar and vanilla.

Combine with the coconut mix, then spoon into individual glasses. Chill until ready to serve.

STEP 2

Peel and chop the kiwi fruit into small pieces. Drain the pineapple, then chop the chunks into small pieces. Mix the fruit together, then spoon over the top of the coconut creams to serve.

Eggs benedict

<u>Ingredients</u>

3 tbsp white wine vinegar

4 eggs

2 toasting muffins

4 parma ham

For the hollandaise sauce

125g butter

2 egg yolks

½ tsp white wine vinegar or tarragon vinegar

squeeze of lemon juice

pinch of cayenne pepper

How to Make

To prepare:

STEP 1

Bring a deep saucepan of water to the boil (at least 2 litres) and add 3 tbsp white wine vinegar. Lower the heat down to a gentle simmer.

STEP 2

Break the eggs into four separate coffee cups or ramekins. Split the muffins, toast them for a few minutes either side and warm some plates.

To make the hollandaise:

STEP 1

Melt the butter in a saucepan and skim any white solids from the surface. Keep the butter warm.

STEP 2

Put the egg yolks, white wine or tarragon vinegar, a pinch of salt and a splash of ice-cold water in a metal or glass bowl that will fit over a small pan. Whisk for a few minutes, then put the bowl over a pan of barely simmering water and whisk continuously until pale and thick, about 3-5 mins.

STEP 3

Remove from the heat and slowly whisk in the melted butter bit by bit until it's all incorporated and you have a creamy hollandaise. (If it gets too thick, add a splash of water.) Season with a squeeze of lemon juice and a little cayenne pepper. Keep warm until needed.

To make the eggs benedict:

STEP 1

Swirl the simmering vinegared water briskly to form a vortex and slide in an egg. It will curl round and set to a neat round shape. Cook for 2-3 mins, then remove with a slotted spoon.

STEP 2

Repeat with the other eggs, one at a time, re-swirling the water as you slide in the eggs. Spread some sauce on each muffin, scrunch a slice of ham on top, then top with an egg. Spoon over the remaining hollandaise and serve at once.

Kale, tomato & poached egg on toast

<u>Ingredients</u>

2 tsp oil

100g ready-chopped kale

1 garlic clove, crushed

½ tsp chilli flakes

2 large eggs

2slices multigrain bread

50g cherry tomatoes, halved

15g feta , crumbled

How to Make

STEP 1

Bring a large pan of water to the boil. Heat the oil in a frying pan over a medium heat and add the kale, garlic and chilli flakes. Cook, stirring occasionally, for 4 mins until the kale begins to crisp and wilt to half its size. Set aside.

STEP 2

Adjust the heat so the water is at a rolling boil, then poach your eggs for 2 mins. Meanwhile, toast the bread.

STEP 3

Remove the poached eggs with a slotted spoon and top each piece of toast with half the kale, an egg, the cherry tomatoes and feta.

Ham & potato hash with baked beans & healthy 'fried' eggs

Ingredients

600g potato, diced

1 Cal cooking spray, for frying

2 leeks, trimmed, washed and sliced

175g lean ham, weighed after trimming and discarding any fat, chopped

2 tbsp wholegrain mustard

5 eggs

2 x 415g cans reduced sugar & salt baked beans

How to Make

STEP 1

Bring a large pan of salted water to the boil. Add the potatoes and boil for 5 mins until just tender. Drain well and leave in the colander to steam-dry.

STEP 2

Meanwhile, spray an ovenproof pan with cooking spray. Add the leeks with a splash of water and fry until very soft and squishy. Add a few more sprays of the oil, tip in the potatoes along with the ham, and fry to crisp up a little. Heat oven to 200C/180C fan/gas 6.

STEP 3

Stir in the mustard, 1 egg and a good amount of seasoning with a fork – break up some of the potatoes roughly as you do. Flatten down the mixture, spray the top with oil, and bake in the oven for 15-20 mins until the top is crisp.

STEP 4

When the hash is nearly ready, heat 200ml water in a non-stick frying pan with a lid (or use a baking sheet as a lid). When it is steaming (but before it simmers), crack in the remaining 4 eggs and cover with a lid. Cook for 2-4 mins until the eggs are done to your liking. Meanwhile, heat the beans.

STEP 5

Lift an egg onto each plate, add a big scoop of hash and spoon on some beans.

Saucy bean baked eggs

Ingredients

2 x 400g cans cherry tomatoes

400g can mixed bean salad, drained

200g baby spinach

4 medium eggs

50g thinly sliced smoked ham, torn

wholemeal rye bread, to serve (optional)

How to Make

STEP 1

Tip the tomatoes and bean salad into an ovenproof frying pan or shallow flameproof casserole dish.

Simmer for 10 mins, or until reduced. Stir in the spinach and cook for 5 mins more until wilted.

STEP 2

Heat the grill to medium. Make four indentations in the mixture using the back of a spoon, then crack one egg in each. Nestle the ham in the mixture, then grill for 4-5 mins, or until the whites are set and the yolks runny. Serve with rye bread, if you like.

Smoky beans on toast

Ingredients

½ tbsp olive oil, plus extra for drizzling

½ small onion, sliced

½ small red pepper, thinly sliced into strips

1 garlic clove, halved

227g can chopped tomatoes

½ tsp smoked paprika

2 tsp red wine vinegar

210g can butter beans or chickpeas, drained

¼ tsp sugar

1 slice seeded bread

a few parsley sprigs, finely chopped

How to Make

STEP 1

Heat the oil in a small pan, add the onion and pepper, and fry gently until soft, about 10-15 mins.

Crush half the garlic and add this to the pan, along with the tomatoes, paprika, vinegar, beans, sugar and some seasoning. Bring to a simmer and cook for 10-15 mins or until slightly reduced and thickened.

STEP 2

Toast the bread, rub with the remaining garlic and drizzle with a little oil. Spoon the beans over the toast, drizzle with a little more oil and scatter over the parsley.

Tofu scramble

Ingredients

1 tbsp olive oil

1 small onion, finely sliced

1 large garlic clove, crushed

½ tsp turmeric

1 tsp ground cumin

½ tsp sweet smoked paprika

280g extra firm tofu

100g cherry tomatoes, halved

½ small bunch parsley, chopped

rye bread, to serve, (optional)

How to Make

STEP 1

Heat the oil in a frying pan over a medium heat and gently fry the onion for 8 -10 mins or until golden brown and sticky. Stir in the garlic, turmeric, cumin and paprika and cook for 1 min.

STEP 2

Roughly mash the tofu in a bowl using a fork, keeping some pieces chunky. Add to the pan and fry for 3 mins. Raise the heat, then tip in the tomatoes, cooking for 5 mins more or until they begin to soften. Fold the parsley through the mixture. Serve on its own or with toasted rye bread (not gluten-free), if you like.

Mushroom baked eggs with squished tomatoes

Ingredients

2 large flat mushrooms (about 85g each), stalks removed and chopped

rapeseed oil, for brushing

½ garlic clove, grated (optional)

a few thyme leaves

2 tomatoes, halved

2 large eggs

2 handfuls rocket

How to Make

STEP 1

Heat oven to 200C/180C fan/gas 6. Brush the mushrooms with a little oil and the garlic (if using). Place the mushrooms in two very lightly greased gratin dishes, bottom-side up, and season lightly with pepper. Top with the chopped stalks and thyme, cover with foil and bake for 20 mins.

STEP 2

Remove the foil, add the tomatoes to the dishes and break an egg carefully onto each of the mushrooms. Season and add a little more thyme, if you like. Return to the oven for 10-12 mins or until the eggs are set but the yolks are still runny. Top with the rocket and eat straight from the dishes.

ESOPHAGITIS-FRIENDLY LUNCH RECIPES

Quick and easy fish stew

<u>Ingredients</u>

1 tbsp olive oil

1 tsp fennel seeds

2 carrots, diced

2 celery sticks, diced

2 garlic cloves, finely chopped

2 leeks, thinly sliced

400g can chopped tomatoes

500ml hot fish stock, heated to a simmer

2 skinless pollock fillets (about 200g), thawed if frozen, and cut into chunks

85g raw shelled king prawns

How to Make

STEP 1

Heat the oil in a large pan, add the fennel seeds, carrots, celery and garlic, and cook for 5 mins until starting to soften. Tip in the leeks, tomatoes and stock, season and bring to the boil, then cover and simmer for 15-20 mins until the vegetables are tender and the sauce has thickened and reduced slightly.

STEP 2

Add the fish, scatter over the prawns and cook for 2 mins more until lightly cooked. Ladle into bowls and serve with a spoon.

Leek, bacon & potato soup

<u>Ingredients</u>

25g butter

3 rashers streaky bacon, chopped

1 onion, chopped

400g pack trimmed leek, sliced and well washed

3 medium potatoes, peeled and diced

1.4l hot vegetable stock,(we used low-sodium)

142ml pot single cream

4 rashers streaky bacon, to serve

<u>How to Make</u>

STEP 1

Melt the butter in a large pan, then fry the bacon and onion, stirring until they start to turn golden. Tip in the leeks and potatoes, stir well, then cover and turn down the heat. Cook gently for 5 mins, shaking the pan every now and then to make sure that the mixture doesn't catch.

STEP 2

Pour in the stock, season well and bring to the boil. Cover and simmer for 20 mins until the vegetables are soft. Leave to cool for a few mins, then blend in a food processor in batches until smooth. Return to the pan, pour in the cream and stir well. Taste and season if necessary. Serve scattered with tasty crisp bacon and eat with toasted or warm crusty bread on the side.

Delicious couscous salad

<u>Ingredients</u>

1 tbsp olive oil

1 tsp fennel seeds

2 carrots, diced

2 celery sticks, diced

2 garlic cloves, finely chopped

2 leeks, thinly sliced

400g can chopped tomatoes

500ml hot fish stock, heated to a simmer

2 skinless pollock fillets (about 200g), thawed if frozen, and cut into chunks

85g raw shelled king prawns

How to Make

STEP 1

Heat the oil in a large pan, add the fennel seeds, carrots, celery and garlic, and cook for 5 mins until starting to soften. Tip in the leeks, tomatoes and stock, season and bring to the boil, then cover and simmer for 15-20 mins until the vegetables are tender and the sauce has thickened and reduced slightly.

STEP 2

Add the fish, scatter over the prawns and cook for 2 mins more until lightly cooked. Ladle into bowls and serve with a spoon

Cauliflower soup

Ingredients

1 large cauliflower (1.5kg), cut into florets

½ tbsp ground cumin

2 tbsp olive oil, plus extra for drizzling

4 thyme sprigs

1 onion, finely chopped

1 celery stick, finely chopped

1 garlic clove, crushed

750-850ml veg or chicken stock

100ml single cream

½ small bunch of parsley, finely chopped

How to Make

STEP 1

Heat the oven to 220C/200C fan/gas 7. Toss the cauliflower florets in a roasting tin with 1 tbsp olive oil, the cumin and the thyme. Roast for 15 mins or until golden and tender. Discard the thyme.

STEP 2

Heat the remaining oil in a saucepan with the onion and celery and fry over a medium heat for 10 mins or until softened. Add the garlic and cook for 1 min.

Stir through most of the cauliflower, reserving some to top the soup with later. Add 750ml of the stock to the pan and bring to a simmer. Cook for 10 mins.

STEP 3

Blitz the soup until smooth using a hand blender or food processor. Stir through the cream and season to taste. Add extra stock if you like your soup a little thinner. Ladle into bowls and top with the parsley, reserved cauliflower and an extra drizzle of olive oil.

Garlic mushrooms

<u>Ingredients</u>

40g butter

500g white mushrooms, or chestnut, halved or quartered; or button chestnut mushrooms kept whole

2 garlic cloves, minced

large handful of parsley leaves, very roughly chopped

How to Make

STEP 1

Melt the butter in a heavy frying pan or skillet over a medium-high heat. When the butter stops sizzling and starts to turn a light brown, throw in the mushrooms and turn the heat up to very high. Season generously with cracked pepper and salt and allow to cook undisturbed for a few mins. No juices should ooze out of the mushrooms; if they do, your pan isn't hot enough and you'll need to turn up the heat to bubble the juices down. Toss the pan and continue to cook all over for 4-5 mins.

STEP 2

With the mushrooms glistening and cooked through, toss through the garlic and cook for 2 mins more. Stir in most of the parsley and leave for another 30 secs. Serve the mushrooms straight from the pan as a side dish, on toast or tossed through spaghetti, with a sprinkling of the remaining parsley.

Prosciutto, kale & butter bean stew

Ingredients

80g pack prosciutto, torn into pieces

2 tbsp olive oil

1 fennel bulb, sliced

2 garlic clove, crushed

1 tsp chilli flakes

4 thyme sprigs

150ml white wine or chicken stock

2 x 400g cans butter beans

400g can cherry tomatoes

200g bag sliced kale

How to Make

STEP 1

Fry the prosciutto in a dry saucepan over a high heat until crisp, then remove half with a slotted spoon and set aside. Turn the heat down to low, pour in the oil and tip in the fennel with a pinch of salt. Cook for 5 mins until softened, then throw in the garlic, chilli flakes and thyme and cook for a further 2 mins, then pour in the wine or stock and bring to a simmer.

STEP 2

Tip both cans of butter beans into the stew, along with their liquid, then add the tomatoes, season well and bring everything to a simmer. Cook, undisturbed, for 5 mins, then stir through the kale. Once wilted, ladle the stew into bowls, removing the thyme sprigs and topping each portion with the remaining prosciutto.

Soup maker mushroom soup

Ingredients

2 medium onions, roughly chopped

1 garlic clove, crushed

500g mushrooms, finely chopped (chestnut or button mushrooms work well)

750ml chicken stock

4 tbsp single cream, plus more to serve

small handful flat-leaf parsley, roughly chopped, to serve (optional)

How to Make

STEP 1

Put the onions, garlic, mushrooms, and stock into the soup maker, and press the 'smooth soup' function. Make sure you don't fill the soup maker above the max fill line.

STEP 2

Once the cycle is complete, season well, and stir in the cream. Blend briefly again until the soup is creamy, then serve in bowls topped with the parsley and more cream if you like.

Cullen skink

<u>Ingredients</u>

1 tbsp unsalted butter

1 medium onion

400g medium potatoes (about 2), peeled and cut into 1cm cubes

250g smoked haddock

250ml whole milk

½ small bunch of parsley or chives, finely chopped

How to Make

STEP 1

Melt the butter in a saucepan over a medium heat, then add the onion and fry for 5-8 mins until translucent but not browned. Add the potatoes and 300ml water and bring to the boil. Reduce the heat slightly and simmer for 10-15 mins.

STEP 2

Meanwhile, put the haddock in another pan and cover with the the milk. Cook gently for 5 mins, or until just tender. Remove the haddock from the milk with a slotted spoon (reserving the milk), transfer to a plate and leave to cool slightly. When cool enough to touch, flake into large pieces, removing any bones.

STEP 3

Put the reserved milk and flaked haddock in the pan with the potato mixture and cook for another 5 mins. Season and sprinkle over the parsley to serve.

Cheat's ramen noodle soup

Ingredients

700ml chicken stock

3 garlic cloves, halved

4 tbsp soy sauce, plus extra to season

1 tsp Worcestershire sauce

thumb-sized piece of ginger, sliced

½ tsp Chinese five spice

pinch of chilli powder

1 tsp white sugar (optional)

375g ramen noodles

400g sliced cooked pork or chicken breast

2 tsp sesame oil

For the garnish

100g baby spinach

4 tbsp sweetcorn

4 boiled eggs, peeled and halved

1 sheet dried nori, finely shredded

sliced green spring onions or shallots

sprinkle of sesame seeds

How to Make

STEP 1

Mix 700ml chicken stock, 3 halved garlic cloves, 4 tbsp soy sauce, 1 tsp Worcestershire sauce, a sliced thumb-sized piece of ginger, ½ tsp Chinese five spice, pinch of chilli powder and 300ml water in a stockpot or large saucepan, bring to the boil, then reduce the heat and simmer for 5 mins.

STEP 2

Taste the stock – add 1 tsp white sugar or a little more soy sauce to make it sweeter or saltier to your liking.

STEP 3

Cook 375g ramen noodles following the pack instructions, then drain and set aside.

STEP 4

Slice 400g cooked pork or chicken, fry in 2 tsp sesame oil until just starting to brown, then set aside.

STEP 5

Divide the noodles between four bowls. Top each with a quarter of the meat, 25g spinach, 1 tbsp sweetcorn and two boiled egg halves each.

STEP 6

Strain the stock into a clean pan, then bring to the boil once again.

STEP 7

Divide the stock between the bowls, then sprinkle over 1 shredded nori sheet, sliced spring onions or shallots and a sprinkle of sesame seeds. Allow the spinach to wilt slightly before serving.

Spiced aubergine bake

<u>Ingredients</u>

4 aubergines, cut into 5mm-1cm slices

3 tbsp vegetable oil

2 tbsp coconut oil

2 large onions, chopped

3 garlic cloves, crushed

1 tbsp black mustard seeds

½ tbsp fenugreek seeds

1 tbsp garam masala

¼ tsp hot chilli powder

1 cinnamon stick

1 tsp ground cumin

1 tsp ground coriander

2 x 400g cans chopped tomatoes

200ml coconut milk

sugar, to taste

2 tbsp flaked almonds

small bunch coriander, roughly chopped (optional)

<u>How to Make</u>

STEP 1

Heat oven to 220C/200C fan/gas 7. Generously brush each aubergine slice with vegetable oil and place in a single layer on a baking tray, or two if they don't fit on one. Cook on the low shelves for 10 mins, then turn over and cook for a further 5-10 mins until they are golden. Reduce the oven to 180C/160C fan/gas 4.

STEP 2

Heat the coconut oil in a large, heavy-based frying pan and add the onions. Cover and sweat on a low heat for about 5 mins until softened. Add the garlic, mustard seeds, fenugreek seeds, garam masala, chilli powder, cinnamon stick, cumin and ground coriander. Cook for a few secs until it starts to smell beautiful and aromatic.

STEP 3

Pour the chopped tomatoes and coconut milk into the spiced onions and stir well. Check the seasoning and add a little sugar, salt or pepper to taste.

STEP 4

Spoon a third of the tomato sauce on the bottom of a 2-litre ovenproof dish. Layer with half the aubergine slices. Spoon over a further third of tomato sauce, then the remaining aubergine slices, and finish with the rest of the sauce. Sprinkle over the flaked almonds and coriander (if using), reserving some to serve, and bake for 25-30 mins. Serve garnished with more coriander.

Speedy lentil coconut curry

<u>Ingredients</u>

1 onion, roughly chopped

2 garlic cloves, roughly chopped

1 red or green chilli, roughly chopped

1 carrot, roughly chopped

10g piece of ginger, peeled and chopped

1 tsp vegetable oil

1 ½ tbsp tikka masala curry paste

400g can cooked green lentils

220ml light coconut milk

200g frozen peas

10g coriander, roughly chopped

200g cooked brown rice

4 tbsp light coconut or natural yogurt, to serve

How to Make

STEP 1

Put the onion, garlic, chilli, carrot and ginger in a food processor and blitz to a smooth paste.

STEP 2

Heat the oil in a medium saucepan over a medium heat and cook the veg paste for 4-5 mins until fragrant and starting to soften. Add the curry paste and cook for 1 min more, then add the lentils and stir to combine.

STEP 3

Pour in the coconut milk and 150ml water, and bring to the boil. Reduce the heat to a simmer and cook for 10 mins until thickened and creamy. Add the peas in the final 5 mins, and season well.

STEP 4

Stir in most of the coriander, then divide the curry between four bowls along with the rice. Sprinkle over the remaining coriander and top with the yogurt to serve.

Summer-in-winter chicken

Ingredients

1 tbsp olive oil

4 boneless skinless chicken breasts

200g pack cherry tomatoes

3 tbsp pesto

3 tbsp crème fraîche (half fat is fine)

fresh basil, if you have it

How to Make

STEP 1

Heat the oil in a frying pan, preferably non-stick. Add the chicken and fry without moving it until it takes on a bit of colour. Turn the chicken and cook on the other side. Continue cooking for 12-15 mins until the chicken is cooked through. Season all over with a little salt and pepper.

STEP 2

Halve the tomatoes and throw them into the pan, stirring them around for a couple of minutes until they start to soften. Reduce the heat and stir in the pesto and crème fraîche until it makes a sauce. Scatter with a few basil leaves if you have them, then serve with rice and salad or mash and broccoli.

Classic Swedish meatballs

<u>Ingredients</u>

400g lean pork mince

1 egg, beaten

1 small onion, finely chopped or grated

85g fresh white breadcrumbs

1 tbsp finely chopped dill, plus extra to serve

1tbsp each olive oil and butter

2 tbsp plain flour

400ml hot beef stock (from a cube is fine)

<u>How to Make</u>

STEP 1

In a bowl, mix the mince with the egg, onion, breadcrumbs, dill and seasoning. Form into small meatballs about the size of walnuts – you should get about 20.

STEP 2

Heat the olive oil in a large non-stick frying pan and brown the meatballs. You may have to do this in 2 batches. Remove from pan, melt the butter, then sprinkle over the flour and stir well. Cook for 2 mins, then slowly whisk in the stock. Keep whisking until it is a thick gravy, then return the meatballs to the pan and heat through. Sprinkle with dill and serve with cranberry jelly, greens and mash.

Bombay potato frittata

<u>Ingredients</u>

4 new potatoes, sliced into 5mm rounds

100g baby spinach, chopped

1 tbsp rapeseed oil

1 onion, halved and sliced

1 large garlic clove, finely grated

½ tsp ground coriander

½ tsp ground cumin

¼ tsp black mustard seeds

¼ tsp turmeric

3 tomatoes, roughly chopped

2 large eggs

½ green chilli, deseeded and finely chopped

1 small bunch of coriander, finely chopped

1 tbsp mango chutney

3 tbsp fat-free Greek yogurt

How to Make

STEP 1

Cook the potatoes in a pan of boiling water for 6 mins, or until tender. Drain and leave to steam-dry. Meanwhile, put the spinach in a heatproof bowl with 1 tbsp water. Cover and microwave for 3 mins on high, or until wilted.

STEP 2

Heat the rapeseed oil in a medium non-stick frying pan. Add the onion and cook over a medium heat for 10 mins until golden and sticky. Stir in the garlic, ground coriander, ground cumin, mustard seeds and turmeric, and cook for 1 min more. Add the tomatoes and wilted spinach and cook for another 3 mins, then add the potatoes.

STEP 3

Heat the grill to medium. Lightly beat the eggs with the chilli and most of the fresh coriander and pour over the potato mixture. Grill for 4-5 mins, or until golden and just set, with a very slight wobble in the middle.

STEP 4

Leave to cool, then slice into wedges. Mix the mango chutney, yogurt and remaining fresh coriander together. Serve with the frittata wedges.

One-pan beef stew with vegetable mash

<u>Ingredients</u>

2 tbsp rapeseed oil

600g pack lean diced beef

320g large chestnut mushrooms, quartered

2 bay leaves

2 tbsp thyme leaves

4 small red onions (320g), quartered

4 garlic cloves, thinly sliced

320g medium carrots, cut into chunky lengths

600ml vegetable stock made with 1 tbsp vegetable bouillon powder

4 tbsp tomato purée

broccoli and/or peas, to serve

For the mash

700g swede, peeled and cut into chunks

850g potatoes, peeled and cut into chunks

How to Make

STEP 1

Heat the oil in a large non-stick pan and fry the beef in about three batches until well browned. Set aside.

STEP 2

Add the mushrooms, bay and thyme to the pan, and cook for about 5 mins. Tip in the onions and garlic, and cook for a few minutes more until softened.

STEP 3

Return the beef to the pan and add the carrots, stock and tomato purée. Cover and simmer for 2 hrs until the meat is tender and the liquid has reduced to a thick gravy.

STEP 4

About 25 mins before the end of the cooking time, make the mash. Bring a large pan of water to the boil and add the swede. Boil for 5 mins, then add the potato and boil for 15-20 mins until tender. Drain and mash with plenty of black pepper.

STEP 5

You can eat half the stew and mash now, then chill the rest to reheat and eat another day. Will keep chilled for a few days. Reheat the stew in a pan until piping hot. The mash can be reheated in the microwave. Serve with broccoli or peas, if you like.

Mushroom brunch

<u>Ingredients</u>

250g mushrooms

1 garlic clove

1 tbsp olive oil

160g bag kale

4 eggs

How to Make

STEP 1

Slice the mushrooms and crush the garlic clove. Heat the olive oil in a large non-stick frying pan, then fry the garlic over a low heat for 1 min. Add the mushrooms and cook until soft. Then, add the kale. If the kale won't all fit in the pan, add half and stir until wilted, then add the rest. Once all the kale is wilted, season.

STEP 2

Now crack in the eggs and keep them cooking gently for 2-3 mins. Then, cover with the lid to for a further 2-3 mins or until the eggs are cooked to your liking. Serve with regular or keto bread for a keto-friendly version.

Chilli chicken wraps

<u>Ingredients</u>

2 tbsp vegetable oil

6 boneless, skinless chicken thighs, cut into bite-sized pieces

1 large onion, thinly sliced into half-moons

2 garlic cloves, finely chopped

3cm piece ginger, peeled and finely chopped

½ tsp ground cumin

½ tsp garam masala

1 tbsp tomato purée

1 red chilli, thinly sliced into rings

juice ½ lemon

4 rotis, warmed

½ small red onion, chopped

4 tbsp mango chutney or lime pickle

4 handfuls mint or coriander

4 tbsp yogurt

How to Make

STEP 1

Heat the oil in a large frying pan over a medium heat. Add the chicken, brown on all sides, then remove. Add the onion, garlic, ginger and a pinch of salt. Cook for 5 mins or until softened.

STEP 2

Increase the heat to high. Return the chicken to the pan with the spices, tomato purée, chilli and lemon juice. Season well and cook for 10 mins or until the chicken is tender.

STEP 3

Divide the chicken, red onion, chutney, herbs and yogurt between the four warm rotis. Roll up and serve with plenty of napkins

Spicy pumpkin soup

Ingredients

127

1 pumpkin, about 1.5-2kg (save the seeds – toast them in a dry pan to serve)

1tbsp garam masala

2tsp ground coriander

2tsp ground cumin

½-1tsp chilli flakes or powder, plus a pinch

3tbsp olive oil

1 onion, finely chopped

ginger, peeled and finely chopped

2 garlic cloves, finely chopped

900ml veg stock

100ml double cream or crème fraiche, plus extra to serve

How to Make

STEP 1

Heat the oven to 180C/160C fan/gas 4. Cut the pumpkin in half and remove the seeds with a spoon (see tip below). Cut into wedges or chunks (keep the skin on) and tip into a bowl. Put the garam masala, and 1 tsp each of the coriander and cumin into a small bowl and mix with 2 tbsp of the oil and season. Drizzle over the pumpkin and toss well to coat in the spiced oil. Transfer to a baking tray, spread out evenly and roast for 40-45 mins, turning halfway through cooking, until the pumpkin is very soft when pierced with a fork. Leave to cool on the tray for a few minutes.

STEP 2

Heat the remaining 1 tbsp olive oil in a large saucepan and fry the onion with a pinch of salt for

10 mins until soft. Add the ginger, garlic and remaining spices and chilli flakes, and fry for a few more minutes until fragrant. Pour in the stock and bring to a gentle simmer.

STEP 3

When the pumpkin is cool enough to touch, use a spoon to scoop the soft flesh from the skins. Add the soft pumpkin to the stock pan, discarding the skins. Remove from the heat and blitz the soup with a hand blender until creamy and smooth. Season to taste, adding extra chilli or garam masala if you like. Put back over a low heat and stir in the cream. Bring to a gentle simmer, then serve in bowls with a drizzle more cream and a pinch of chilli to serve. Top with toasted pumpkin seeds, if you like.

ESOPHAGITIS-FRIENDLY DINNER RECIPES

Delicious Pumpkin masala

<u>Ingredients</u>

1 pumpkin, about 1.5-2kg (save the seeds – toast them in a dry pan to serve)

1tbsp garam masala

2tsp ground coriander

2tsp ground cumin

½-1tsp chilli flakes or powder, plus a pinch

3tbsp olive oil

1 onion, finely chopped

ginger, peeled and finely chopped

2 garlic cloves, finely chopped

900ml veg stock

100ml double cream or crème fraiche, plus extra to serve

How to Make

STEP 1

Heat the oven to 180C/160C fan/gas 4. Cut the pumpkin in half and remove the seeds with a spoon (see tip below). Cut into wedges or chunks (keep the skin on) and tip into a bowl. Put the garam masala, and 1 tsp each of the coriander and cumin into a small bowl and mix with 2 tbsp of the oil and season. Drizzle over the pumpkin and toss well to coat in the spiced oil. Transfer to a baking tray, spread out evenly and roast for 40-45 mins, turning halfway through cooking, until the pumpkin is very soft when pierced with a fork. Leave to cool on the tray for a few minutes.

STEP 2

Heat the remaining 1 tbsp olive oil in a large saucepan and fry the onion with a pinch of salt for 10 mins until soft. Add the ginger, garlic and remaining spices and chilli flakes, and fry for a few more minutes until fragrant. Pour in the stock and bring to a gentle simmer.

STEP 3

When the pumpkin is cool enough to touch, use a spoon to scoop the soft flesh from the skins. Add the soft pumpkin to the stock pan, discarding the skins. Remove from the heat and blitz the soup with a hand blender until creamy and smooth. Season to taste, adding extra chilli or garam masala if you like. Put back over a low heat and stir in the cream. Bring to a gentle simmer, then serve in bowls with a drizzle more cream and a pinch of chilli to serve. Top with toasted pumpkin seeds, if you like.

Cajun chicken pasta

<u>Ingredients</u>

1 tbsp olive oil

400g chicken breasts, chopped into large chunks

3 garlic cloves, finely chopped or grated

2 tbsp Cajun-style seasoning

400g can chopped tomatoes or passata

1 chicken stock cube, crumbled

500g penne or another tube- shaped pasta

150ml double cream

20g parmesan, finely grated, plus extra to serve

½ lemon, juiced

chopped parsley, to serve (optional)

<u>How to Make</u>

STEP 1

Heat the olive oil in a large, shallow saucepan or deep frying pan over a medium heat, then add the chicken, season lightly and fry for 6-8 mins, stirring occasionally until just golden all over – no need to worry about it being cooked through at this stage.

STEP 2

Stir in the garlic and cook for 2 mins more, then scatter over the Cajun-style seasoning and stir so the chicken pieces are evenly coated. Tip in the tomatoes, a quarter of a can of water and the stock cube. Stir, then bring to a simmer and cook for 5 mins.

STEP 3

Meanwhile, bring a large pan of salted water to the boil and cook the pasta for a minute less than pack instructions. Stir the cream into the chicken and continue to simmer gently. When the pasta is cooked, drain well and stir into chicken mixture. Finish cooking the pasta in the sauce over a low heat for 2 mins, then stir in the parmesan and lemon juice, and cook for 1 min more. Serve the pasta straight from the pan, or tip into a large serving bowl. Scatter with parsley, if you like, and extra parmesan.

Mushroom risotto

Ingredients

50g dried porcini mushrooms

1 vegetable stock cube

2 tbsp olive oil

1 onion, finely chopped

2 garlic cloves, finely chopped

250g pack chestnut mushrooms, chopped

300g risotto rice, such as arborio

1 x 175ml glass white wine

25g butter

handful parsley leaves, chopped

50g parmesan or Grana Padano, freshly grated

How to Make

STEP 1

Put 50g dried porcini mushrooms into a large bowl and pour over 1 litre boiling water. Soak for 20 mins, then drain into a bowl, discarding the last few tbsp of liquid left in the bowl.

STEP 2

Crumble 1 vegetable stock cube into the mushroom liquid, then squeeze the mushrooms gently to remove any liquid.

STEP 3

Heat 2 tbsp olive oil in a shallow saucepan or deep frying pan over a medium flame. Add 1 finely chopped onion and 2 finely chopped garlic cloves, then fry for about 5 mins until soft.

STEP 4

Stir in 250g chopped chestnut mushrooms and the dried mushrooms, season with salt and pepper and continue to cook for 8 mins until the fresh mushrooms have softened.

STEP 5

Tip 300g risotto rice into the pan and cook for 1 min. Pour over a 175ml glass of white wine and let it bubble to nothing so the alcohol evaporates.

STEP 6

Keep the pan over a medium heat and pour in a quarter of the mushroom stock. Simmer the rice, stirring often, until the rice has absorbed all the liquid.

STEP 7

Add about the same amount of stock again and continue to simmer and stir - it should start to become creamy, plump and tender. By the time the final quarter of stock is added, the rice should be almost cooked.

STEP 8

Continue stirring until the rice is cooked. If the rice is still undercooked, add a splash of water. Take the pan off the heat, add 25g butter and scatter over 25g grated parmesan or Grana Padano cheese and half a handful of chopped parsley leaves.

STEP 9

Cover and leave for a few mins so that the rice can take up any excess liquid as it cools a bit. Give the risotto a final stir, spoon into bowls and scatter with the remaining 25g grated cheese and the remaining chopped parsley leaves.

Honey chicken

Ingredients

4 chicken breasts (about 600g), trimmed and cut into 2-3cm cubes

2 tbsp plain flour

40g piece of ginger, peeled and finely grated

4 garlic cloves, finely chopped

6 tbsp soy sauce

5 tbsp honey

½-1 lemon, juiced

1 tbsp sunflower, vegetable, rice bran or rapeseed oil

cooked rice and steamed broccoli, to serve (optional)

<u>How to Make</u>

STEP 1

Tip the chicken into a bowl, sprinkle over the flour and some seasoning and toss until the chicken is evenly coated.

STEP 2

Combine the ginger, garlic, soy, honey and half the lemon juice in a bowl. Heat the oil in a large frying pan or wok over a high heat and fry the chicken for 3-4 mins until lightly golden. Tip in the honey sauce and stir-fry for 10 mins, or until the chicken is cooked through and the sauce has reduced enough to coat the back of a spoon. Taste for seasoning and squeeze over the remaining lemon juice, if needed, then serve with rice and steamed broccoli, if you like.

Slow cooker pork casserole

Ingredients

1 tbsp vegetable or rapeseed oil

4 pork shoulder steaks (about 750g), cut into large
chunks

1 onion, chopped

1 leek, chopped

1 carrot, chopped

bundle of woody herbs (bouquet garni) – we used 2
bay leaves, 3 sage leaves and 4 thyme sprigs, plus a
few thyme leaves to serve

1 chicken stock cube

2 tsp Dijon mustard

1 tbsp cider vinegar

2 tsp cornflour

1 tbsp honey

How to Make

STEP 1

Heat your slow cooker. Drizzle the oil in a wide frying pan over a high heat. Season the pork, then add to the hot pan. Avoid overcrowding the meat – you may want to do this in batches. Cook until deep brown all over, then transfer to the slow cooker. Add the onion and leeks to the frying pan and cook for a few mins, until they soften. Add a splash of water and scrape any tasty bits from the bottom, then tip everything into the slow cooker. Add the carrot, herbs, stock cube, mustard and vinegar, season, then add enough water to just cover the ingredients. Stir, then set your slow cooker on low for 6-8 hrs, or high for 5-6 hrs.

STEP 2

In a saucepan, mix the cornflour and honey with 1-2 tsp of liquid from the slow cooker, until you have a smooth paste. Add 100ml more liquid, bring to a simmer until thickened, then stir back into the casserole. Serve with mash or dumplings, scattered with thyme leaves.

Tuna, caper & chilli spaghetti

<u>Ingredients</u>

150g spaghetti or linguine

1 tbsp olive oil

1 garlic clove, sliced

1 red chilli, deseeded and finely chopped, plus extra to serve (optional)

1 tbsp drained capers

small bunch of parsley, finely chopped (stalks included)

145g tuna in spring water, drained

90g rocket or baby spinach leaves

½ lemon, juiced

How to Make

STEP 1

Cook the spaghetti for 9-11 mins in a large pan of well-salted water until al dente.

STEP 2

Heat the oil in a wide frying pan over a very low heat, and gently cook the garlic and chilli to infuse the oil. Remove from the heat if the garlic is turning past light golden, as this will make it bitter.

STEP 3

Drain the pasta, keeping a cupful of the cooking water, and tip the spaghetti into the frying pan. Toss the pasta in the oil over a low heat, adding a little of the pasta water to emulsify into a sauce that coats the pasta, then fold in the capers, parsley, tuna and some seasoning. Don't stir too vigorously – you want to keep larger chunks of tuna. Toss the rocket and lemon juice through the spaghetti, and serve with extra chilli scattered over, if you like

Beetroot risotto with feta

Ingredients

2 tbsp olive oil, plus extra to serve

1 onion, finely chopped

300g raw beetroot, grated

1 garlic clove, crushed

175g risotto rice

100ml white wine

600ml hot vegetable stock

50g grated parmesan or vegetarian alternative

½ lemon, zested and juiced

40g feta, crumbled

small handful of dill, to serve (optional)

How to Make

STEP 1

Heat the oil in a large saucepan. Add the onion and beetroot, and cook over a low-medium heat for 15 mins. Add the garlic and cook for 1 min. Stir in the rice and fry for a couple of minutes, then pour in the wine and bring to a simmer. Add half the stock, stirring until it is absorbed. Add the remaining stock, a ladleful at a time, stirring continuously until the rice is al dente. Stir through the parmesan and lemon juice, adding a splash more stock to loosen if the risotto seems a little thick. Season to taste.

STEP 2

Toss the feta with the lemon zest and dill, if using, and spoon over the risotto. Finish with a drizzle of olive oil. Any leftovers will keep covered in the fridge for up to three days. Reheat in a pan over a low heat, stirring in a little stock to loosen.

Slow cooker pulled chicken

<u>Ingredients</u>

2 tbsp vegetable or rapeseed oil

10-12 boneless, skinless chicken thighs

2 red onions, halved and sliced

2 garlic cloves, crushed

2 tsp paprika

2 tbsp chipotle paste

250ml passata

100g barbecue sauce

1 tbsp light brown soft sugar

1 lime, juiced

burger buns, taco shells, jacket potatoes or rice; coriander leaves; deseeded and sliced chillies, and guacamole, to serve (optional)

How to Make

STEP 1

Heat the slow cooker to low and heat 1 tbsp oil in a pan. Brown the chicken in batches, transferring it to the slow cooker as you go. Add the remaining oil to the pan and fry the onions for 5 mins, or until just softened, then stir in the garlic and paprika and cook for another minute. Tip into the slow cooker, then swirl 100ml water around the pan and pour this in as well.

STEP 2

Add the chipotle, passata, barbecue sauce, sugar and lime juice, then season and stir. Cover and cook for 6-8 hrs until the chicken is really tender. Using two forks, shred the chicken through the sauce. Serve in buns, taco shells, jacket potatoes or over rice, with coriander leaves, chillies and guacamole, if you like.

Creamy mushroom & spinach pasta

<u>Ingredients</u>

2 tbsp olive oil

1 small onion, finely chopped

150g baby mushrooms, halved

150g tagliatelle

2 garlic cloves, crushed

200g low-fat crème fraîche

15g parmesan or vegetarian alternative, grated

120g baby spinach

½ tsp chilli flakes (optional)

How to Make

STEP 1

Heat the oil in a medium saucepan over a medium heat and fry the onion and mushrooms for 10 mins, or until softened and browned slightly. Meanwhile, cook the pasta following pack instructions.

STEP 2

Add the garlic to the pan with the mushrooms and cook for 2 mins more. Tip in the crème fraîche and parmesan, stir to combine, then add the baby spinach. Set aside.

STEP 3

Remove the pasta from the heat and drain, reserving 25ml of the water. Toss the pasta in the creamy mushroom sauce, put back on the heat and cook over a low heat until the spinach wilts, about 5 mins. Pour in enough of the reserved water to loosen slightly. Season with black pepper and finish with a sprinkle of chilli flakes, if you like.

Mushroom & potato curry

Ingredients

1 tbsp oil

1 onion, roughly chopped

1 large potato, chopped into small chunks

1 aubergine, trimmed and chopped into chunks

250g button mushrooms

2-4 tbsp curry paste (depending on how hot you like it)

150ml vegetable stock

400ml can reduced-fat coconut milk

chopped coriander, to serve

How to Make

STEP 1

Heat the oil in a large saucepan, add the onion and potato. Cover, then cook over a low heat for 5 mins until the potatoes start to soften. Throw in the aubergine and mushrooms, then cook for a few more mins.

STEP 2

Stir in the curry paste, pour over the stock and coconut milk. Bring to the boil, then simmer for 10 mins or until the potato is tender. Stir through the coriander and serve with rice or naan bread.

Prawn jambalaya

<u>Ingredients</u>

1 tbsp rapeseed oil

1 onion, chopped

3 celery sticks, sliced

100g wholegrain basmati rice

1 tsp mild chilli powder

1 tbsp ground coriander

½ tsp fennel seeds

400g can chopped tomatoes

1 tsp vegetable bouillon powder

1 yellow pepper, roughly chopped

2 garlic cloves, chopped

1 tbsp fresh thyme leaves

150g pack small prawns, thawed if frozen

3 tbsp chopped parsley

How to Make

STEP 1

Heat the oil in a large, deep frying pan. Add the onion and celery, and fry for 5 mins to soften. Add the rice and spices, and pour in the tomatoes with just under 1 can of water. Stir in the bouillon powder, pepper, garlic and thyme.

STEP 2

Cover the pan with a lid and simmer for 30 mins until the rice is tender and almost all the liquid has been absorbed. Stir in the prawns and parsley, cook briefly to heat through, then serve.

Tomato & spinach kitchari

<u>Ingredients</u>

130g basmati rice

200g split red lentils

3 tbsp olive oil

1 onion, finely sliced

1 thumb-sized piece ginger, finely grated

2 garlic cloves, crushed

2 tsp turmeric

2 tsp ground coriander

2 tsp cumin seeds

1-2 tsp medium chilli powder

1.2l vegetable stock

150g cherry tomatoes

200g spinach

1 red chilli, finely chopped

chapatis, to serve (optional)

How to Make

STEP 1

Tip the rice and lentils into a sieve and rinse thoroughly under cold, running water. Set aside.

STEP 2

Heat 1 tbsp of the oil in a large saucepan or casserole. Add the onion along with a pinch of salt and fry over a medium-high heat for 10 mins or until golden. Stir through the ginger, garlic, turmeric, ground coriander, half the cumin seeds and the chilli powder and fry for 1 min. Add the rice and lentils to the pan and pour in the stock, bring to a simmer then cover, turn down and cook for 25 mins, stirring now and then, until the lentils have turned creamy. Add the tomatoes and spinach and cook for 5 mins.

STEP 3

Heat the remaining oil in a small frying pan and add the remaining cumin seeds, cooking for 1 min. Spoon the lentils into four bowls, drizzle over the cumin oil and top with the chilli. Serve with warm chapatis, if you like

Slow cooker gammon in cola

<u>Ingredients</u>

1.5-1.8kg unsmoked boneless gammon joint

2l cola (not diet)

1 carrot, peeled and chopped

1 onion, peeled and quartered

1 stick celery, chopped

1 cinnamon stick

½ tbsp peppercorns

1 bay leaf

For the glaze

150ml maple syrup

2 tbsp wholegrain mustard

2 tbsp red wine vinegar

pinch of ground cloves or five-spice

How to Make

STEP 1

Set your slow cooker to medium. Place the gammon joint in and cover with the cola. Add 1 chopped carrot, 1 quartered onion, 1 chopped celery stick, 1 cinnamon stick, ½ tbsp peppercorns and 1 bay leaf.

STEP 2

Cook for 5½ hrs on low until the gammon is tender but still holding its shape, topping up with boiling water if necessary to keep the gammon fully covered.

STEP 3

Carefully pour the liquid away, then let the ham cool a little while you heat the oven to 190C/170C fan/gas 5. Lift the ham into a roasting tin, then cut away the skin leaving behind an even layer of fat. Score the fat all over in a criss-cross pattern.

STEP 4

Mix the maple syrup, mustard, vinegar and ground cloves or five-spice in a jug. Pour half over the fat, roast for 15 mins, then pour over the rest and return to the oven for another 30 mins.

STEP 5

Remove from the oven and allow to rest for 10 mins, then spoon more glaze over the top. Can be roasted on the day or up to two days ahead and served cold.

Tomato & thyme cod

Ingredients

1 tbsp olive oil

1 onion, chopped

400g can chopped tomatoes

1 heaped tsp light soft brown sugar

few sprigs thyme, leaves stripped

1 tbsp soy sauce

4 cod fillets, or another white flaky fish, such as pollock

How to Make

STEP 1

Heat 1 tbsp olive oil in a frying pan, add 1 chopped onion, then fry for 5-8 mins until lightly browned.

STEP 2

Stir in a 400g can chopped tomatoes, 1 heaped tsp light soft brown sugar, the leaves from a few sprigs of thyme and 1 tbsp soy sauce, then bring to the boil.

STEP 3

Simmer 5 mins, then slip 4 cod fillets into the sauce.

STEP 4

Cover and gently cook for 8-10 mins until the cod flakes easily. Serve with baked or steamed potatoes.

Katsu curry

Ingredients

4 tbsp rapeseed oil or vegetable oil

2 x 200g pouches cooked rice (we used brown basmati)

½ large cucumber, peeled into ribbons

handful mint leaves or coriander leaves, or both

lime wedges, to serve

For the curry sauce

1 tbsp rapeseed oil or vegetable oil

2 onions, chopped

2 large carrots, chopped, plus 1 peeled into ribbons

2 garlic cloves, crushed

thumb-sized piece ginger, peeled and grated or finely chopped

1 tbsp curry powder, mild or medium depending on your spice tolerance

½ tsp ground turmeric

400ml can coconut milk

2 tsp maple syrup (or use honey if not cooking for vegans)

For the katsu

1 tbsp cornflour

8 chicken mini fillets, or a 280-300g block firm tofu, or half and half

200g breadcrumbs (gluten-free if necessary)

How to Make

STEP 1

First, make the curry sauce. Heat 1 tbsp oil in a pan, cook the onions and chopped carrots until the onions are soft and starting to caramelise, about 8 mins. Add the garlic and ginger and sizzle for another 30 secs, then stir in the curry powder and turmeric. Once the spices are warmed through, add the coconut milk, maple syrup or honey and 100ml water. Season well, cover and simmer over a low heat for 20 mins.

STEP 2

Now make the katsu. In a wide bowl, mix the cornflour with 4 tbsp water and some seasoning. Dip the chicken or tofu into the flour mixture (if cooking for both vegans and meat eaters, make sure you dip the tofu first to avoid mixing it with meat).

Place the breadcrumbs in another bowl and dip the chicken or tofu in it, turning until well coated.

STEP 3

When the onions and carrots in the curry sauce are soft, blitz using a hand or table-top blender. If the sauce is too thick, add a little more water, check the seasoning, adding more salt, maple syrup or some lime juice, if you like. Keep warm.

STEP 4

Heat the oil in a frying pan and cook the chicken or tofu for 4-5 mins on each side until golden and cooked through. Warm the rice and divide between bowls. Top with the curry sauce, katsu chicken or tofu, and serve with the cucumber, carrot ribbons, herbs and lime wedges.

Slow cooker vegetable lasagne

<u>Ingredients</u>

1 tbsp rapeseed oil

2 onions, sliced

2 large garlic cloves, chopped

2 large courgettes, diced (400g)

1 red and 1 yellow pepper, deseeded and roughly sliced

400g can chopped tomatoes

2 tbsp tomato purée

2 tsp vegetable bouillon

15g fresh basil, chopped plus a few leaves

1 large aubergine, sliced across length or width for maximum surface area

6 wholewheat lasagne sheets (105g)

125g vegetarian buffalo mozzarella, chopped

How to Make

STEP 1

Heat 1 tbsp rapeseed oil in a large non-stick pan and fry 2 sliced onions and 2 chopped large garlic cloves for 5 mins, stirring frequently until softened.

STEP 2

Tip in 2 diced large courgettes, 1 red and 1 yellow pepper, both roughly sliced, and 400g chopped tomatoes with 2 tbsp tomato purée, 2 tsp vegetable bouillon and 15g chopped basil.

STEP 3

Stir well, cover and cook for 5 mins. Don't be tempted to add more liquid as plenty of moisture will come from the vegetables once they start cooking.

STEP 4

Slice 1 large aubergine. Lay half the slices of aubergine in the base of the slow cooker and top with 3 sheets of lasagne.

STEP 5

Add a third of the ratatouille mixture, then the remaining aubergine slices, 3 more lasagne sheets, then the remaining ratatouille mixture.

STEP 6

Cover and cook on High for 2½ - 3 hours until the pasta and vegetables are tender. Turn off the machine.

STEP 7

Scatter 125g vegetarian buffalo mozzarella over the vegetables then cover and leave for 10 mins to settle and melt the cheese.

STEP 8

Scatter with extra basil and serve with a handful of rocket.

Harissa-crumbed fish with lentils & peppers

Ingredients

2 x 200g pouches cooked puy lentils

200g jar roasted red peppers, drained and torn into chunks

50g black olives, from a jar, roughly chopped

1 lemon, zested and cut into wedges

3 tbsp olive or rapeseed oil

4 x 140g cod fillets (or another white fish)

100g fresh breadcrumbs

1 tbsp harissa

½ small pack flat-leaf parsley, chopped

How to Make

STEP 1

Heat oven to 200C/180C fan/gas 6. Mix the lentils, peppers, olives, lemon zest, 2 tbsp oil and some seasoning in a roasting tin. Top with the fish fillets. Mix the breadcrumbs, harissa and the remaining oil and put a few spoonfuls on top of each piece of fish. Bake for 12-15 mins until the fish is cooked, the topping is crispy and the lentils are hot. Scatter with the parsley and squeeze over the lemon wedges.

ESOPHAGITIS-FRIENDLY DESSERTS

Apple, cream & spiced rye crumble pots

<u>Ingredients</u>

4 cooking apples

6 tbsp caster sugar

50g unsalted butter

100g brown breadcrumbs

100g soft light brown sugar

½ tsp cinnamon

ground cardamom from 8 cardamom pods

100g rye breadcrumbs

500ml whipping cream

5 tbsp icing sugar (or add to taste)

good squeeze of lemon

2 tbsp aquavit (optional), or to taste

2 tbsp blanched hazelnuts, halved and toasted

How to Make

STEP 1

Peel and core the apples and cut the flesh into chunks. Put these in a large saucepan with the caster sugar and 3 tbsp water and cook over a gentle heat until the apples are completely tender. Stir every so often and mash the fruit down roughly with the back of a wooden spoon. The finished purée shouldn't be too wet – if it is, simmer it over a low heat until it reduces and loses some of its moisture.

STEP 2

Check the apples for sweetness – they shouldn't be too sweet as it's being mixed with sweet cream and breadcrumbs – and tip into a bowl to cool. In Scandinavia, the stewed apples are usually puréed until smooth, but you can also keep them chunky.

STEP 3

Melt half the butter in a frying pan and add the brown breadcrumbs and half the brown sugar. Sauté, stirring constantly, over a medium heat until the breadcrumbs are golden. Add half the cinnamon and half the cardamom and continue to cook for about 1 min. Spread out on a tray – it cools quicker this way – and leave until it's room temperature. Do the same with the rye breadcrumbs, then mix the breadcrumbs together in a bowl.

Key lime pie

<u>Ingredients</u>

300g oatmeal biscuits

110g butter, melted

1 x 397g can condensed milk (we used Nestlé)

3 medium egg yolks

finely grated zest and juice of 4 limes

300ml double cream

1 tbsp icing sugar

extra lime zest, to decorate

<u>How to Make</u>

STEP 1

Heat the oven to 160C/fan 140C/gas 3.

STEP 2

Whizz 300g oatmeal biscuits to crumbs in a food processor (or put in a strong plastic bag and bash with a rolling pin).

STEP 3

Mix with 110g melted butter and press into the base and up the sides of a 22cm loose-based tart tin. Bake in the oven for 10 minutes. Remove and cool.

STEP 4

Put 3 medium egg yolks in a large bowl and whisk for a minute with electric beaters.

STEP 5

Add a can of condensed milk and whisk for 3 minutes, then add the finely grated zest and juice of 4 limes and whisk again for 3 minutes.

STEP 6

Pour the filling into the cooled base then put back in the oven for 15 minutes. Cool then chill for at least 6 hours or overnight if you like. When you are ready to serve, carefully remove the pie from the tin and put on a serving plate.

STEP 7

To decorate, softly whip together 300ml double cream and 1 tbsp icing sugar.

STEP 8

Dollop or pipe the cream onto the top of the pie and finish with extra lime zest.

Pumpkin bread

Ingredients

175g butter, melted

140g clear honey

1 large egg, beaten

250g raw peeled pumpkin, or butternut squash, coarsely grated (about 500g/1lb 2oz before peeling and seeding)

100g light muscovado sugar

350g self-raising flour

1 tbsp ground ginger

2 tbsp demerara sugar

<u>How to Make</u>

STEP 1

Preheat the oven to 180C/gas 4/ fan 160C. Butter and line the base and two long sides of a 1.5kg loaf tin with a strip of baking paper.

STEP 2

Mix the butter, honey and egg and stir in the pumpkin or squash. Then mix in the sugar, flour and ginger.

STEP 3

Pour into the prepared tin and sprinkle the top with the demerara sugar. Bake for 50-60 minutes, until risen and golden brown. Leave in the tin for 5 minutes, then turn out and cool on a wire rack. Serve thickly sliced and buttered.

Slow cooker sticky toffee pudding

<u>Ingredients</u>

250g pitted dates, chopped

100g butter, plus extra for the basin

4 tbsp treacle

1 tsp vanilla extract

250g light brown soft sugar

300ml double cream

2 eggs, lightly beaten

200g self-raising flour

1 tsp bicarbonate of soda

vanilla ice cream, to serve

How to Make

STEP 1

Put the dates in a heatproof bowl, cover with 150ml boiling water, and leave to soak for 30 mins. Butter a 1-litre pudding basin and line the base with baking parchment.

STEP 2

Tip half the butter, half the treacle, the vanilla, 75g of the sugar and the cream into a pan set over a medium heat. Cook for 4-5 mins, stirring, until the sugar dissolves. Turn up the heat, bubble for 3 mins, then whisk in a pinch of salt. Pour a third of the sauce into the basin.

STEP 3

Beat the remaining butter, treacle, sugar and the eggs together, then fold in the flour, bicarb, ¼ tsp salt, the dates and their soaking liquid. Spoon into the basin and smooth the surface, leaving a 1cm gap from the top. Cover with a double layer of baking parchment and foil, making a pleat in the middle so the pud can expand. Secure with kitchen string.

STEP 4

Set the slow cooker to low. Sit the basin inside, then add boiling water so it comes halfway up the basin. Cover and cook for 7-8 hrs. Run a knife around the edge of the pudding and turn out onto a plate.

Reheat the remaining sauce and pour over. Serve with ice cream.

Poached pears in red wine

<u>Ingredients</u>

1 vanilla pod

1 bottle red wine

225g caster sugar

1 cinnamon stick, halved

fresh thyme sprig, plus sprigs to seve

6 pears, peeled, but kept whole with stalk intact

<u>How to Make</u>

STEP 1

Halve the vanilla pod lengthways, scrape out the black seeds and put in a large saucepan with the wine, sugar, cinnamon and thyme. Cut each piece of pod into three long thin strips, add to pan, then lower in the pears.

STEP 2

Poach the pears, covered, for 20-30 mins, making sure they are covered in the wine. The cooking time will very much depend on the ripeness of your pears – they should be tender all the way through when pierced with a cocktail stick. You can make these up to 2 days ahead and chill.

STEP 3

Take the pears from the pan, then boil the liquid to reduce it by half so that it's syrupy. Serve each pear with the cooled syrup, a strip of vanilla, a piece of cinnamon and a small thyme sprig.

Profiteroles

<u>Ingredients</u>

50g butter (preferably unsalted), cut into cubes

2 tbsp caster sugar

75g strong white flour, sifted with a pinch of fine sea salt

2 eggs, lightly beaten

300ml double cream

few drops vanilla extract

For the sauce

50g cocoa powder

175g caster sugar

How to Make

STEP 1

Heat the oven to 220C/200C fan/gas 7. To make the profiteroles, put the butter and 2 tsp of the caster sugar in a saucepan with 150ml water. Place the pan over a low heat until the butter and sugar have melted, then bring to the boil. Take off the heat, add the flour all at once and beat energetically with a wooden spoon until the dough comes away from the sides of the pan.

STEP 2

Leave to cool for 5 mins, then beat in the eggs bit by bit until you have a stiff, glossy mixture (this process is much easier in a food processor). Rinse two baking trays with cold water, shaking off any excess so they are slightly damp (this helps the pastry to rise). Using 2 teaspoons, spoon blobs of the mixture onto the baking trays. Then place in the oven and cook for about 18-20 mins until well risen and brown. Remove the profiteroles from the oven and cut a small slit in the base of each one so they don't collapse. Cool on a wire rack.

STEP 3

When they're cold, whip the cream lightly until just holding its shape. Sweeten to taste with remaining sugar and a few drops of vanilla extract. Cut the profiteroles in half, fill them with the sweetened cream and pile them up on a plate. You can refrigerate them for 1-2 hrs at this point but not for any longer as the pastry will go soggy.

STEP 4

To make the sauce, sift the cocoa powder into a bowl. Put the sugar in a pan with 100ml water and warm over a low heat until dissolved. Bring to the boil, cook for 1 min, then pour over the cocoa powder and stir well until smooth. Return the sauce to the pan, cook for 1 min then set aside for 15 mins before drizzling over the profiteroles.

Marmalade muffins

<u>Ingredients</u>

175g plain flour

25g porridge oat, plus extra for sprinkling

175g light soft brown sugar

1 tsp baking powder

½ tsp bicarbonate of soda

zest and juice 1 orange

1 tbsp sunflower oil

150g pot plain yogurt

1 large egg

9 tsp chunky marmalade

How to Make

STEP 1

Heat oven to 200C/180C fan/ gas 6 and line a muffin tin with 9 paper cases. Combine the flour, oats, sugar, baking powder and bicarb in a bowl. Whisk the orange zest and juice, oil, yogurt and egg together with a fork, then lightly stir the 2 mixtures together until just combined.

STEP 2

Spoon 1 tbsp of the mixture into each muffin case, top with 1 tsp of marmalade, then cover with the remaining muffin mix and a sprinkling of oats. Bake for 15-20 mins until cooked through and golden, then leave to cool slightly.

Rhubarb & ginger crème brûlée

Ingredients

400g forced rhubarb, chopped into 3cm pieces

40g caster sugar

4 balls stem ginger in syrup, chopped

2 tsp cornflour

For the custard layer

500ml double cream

150g caster sugar

1 vanilla pod, split lengthways

3 large eggs

5 tbsp demerara sugar

How to Make

STEP 1

Put the rhubarb in a pan with the sugar and chopped ginger. Cook over a low heat for 10 mins or until the rhubarb has softened and begun to break down. Mix a little of the rhubarb juice with the cornflour in a small bowl, then pour into the pan and stir until thickened. Pour into the base of a round roughly 20cm dish. Leave to cool completely.

STEP 2

For the custard, pour the double cream, sugar and vanilla pod (as well as the scraped-out seeds) into a pan and bring to a simmer. Scoop out the pod and discard. Whisk the eggs in a bowl and gradually pour over the simmering cream, whisking continuously. Pour the mixture back into the pan. Cook over a low heat, continuously stirring, for around 10 mins until it reaches 86C on a cooking thermometer, or is thickened. Pour over the cooled rhubarb, smooth to an even layer and chill overnight.

STEP 3

Sprinkle the demerara sugar over the top and caramelise using a blowtorch until deep golden brown. Serve.

Coconut, rum & raisin rice pudding

<u>Ingredients</u>

50g butter

150g short-grain pudding rice

150g golden caster sugar

2 x 400ml cans coconut milk

300ml double cream, plus a little extra

1 tsp vanilla extract

For the rum & raisin syrup

150ml spiced rum

100g muscovado sugar

100g raisins

How to Make

STEP 1

For the rum & raisin syrup, tip all the ingredients into a large saucepan and heat gently over a low heat for 5 mins, or until the sugar has dissolved and created a syrup and the raisins have plumped up. Tip into a bowl, cover and set aside.

STEP 2

In the same saucepan (there's no need to clean it) melt the butter over a medium heat until sizzling, then scatter over the rice and toast in the hot butter until the butter is just starting to brown. Stir in the sugar, then pour over the coconut milk, cream and vanilla. Bring to a simmer and continue to cook gently for 40-45 mins until the rice is tender, adding a splash more cream if it becomes too thick.

STEP 3

To serve hot, stir a third of the rum & raisin syrup through the pudding and spoon the rest over the top. To serve cold, leave the pudding to cool, then chill in the fridge to firm up so that you can serve it in scoops with the rum & raisin syrup spooned over.

French apple tart

<u>Ingredients</u>

For the pastry

125g cold butter, cubed

200g plain flour, plus extra for dusting

1 tbsp golden caster sugar

1 egg, beaten

For the filling and topping

1 ¾ kg (about 12) eating apples, like Cox's, Russet or Granny Smith

50g golden caster sugar

1 tbsp calvados, cognac or brandy (optional)

25g butter, melted

3 tbsp apricot jam

icing sugar, to serve (optional)

How to Make

STEP 1

For the pastry, rub the butter into the flour, sugar and a pinch of salt in a bowl until crumbly. Mix in the egg until it forms a dough, then form into a puck shape. Cover and chill for at least 30 mins. Will keep chilled for two days.

STEP 2

Heat the oven to 200C/180C fan/ gas 6. Roll the pastry out on a lightly floured surface to roughly the thickness of a £1 coin, and use to line a 23cm fluted tart tin, leaving some overhanging. Line with a disc of baking parchment big enough to cover the edges, and fill with some baking beans to weigh it down (use dried rice or lentils if you don't have baking beans). Bake for 15 mins, then remove the parchment and beans and bake for 10-15 mins more until the pastry is biscuity. Trim away any overhanging pastry with a serrated knife. Set aside to cool.

STEP 3

Meanwhile, set aside four of the apples, then peel, core and roughly chop the rest. Put them in a shallow saucepan with 2 tbsp water, all but 1 tbsp of the sugar and the alcohol, if using. Cover and cook over a low heat for 25-30 mins, stirring occasionally and adding more water if needed, until the apples have collapsed into a purée. Taste the mixture and sweeten with more sugar, if needed.

STEP 4

Turn the oven up to 210C/190C fan/gas 8. Peel, core and halve the reserved apples, then cut into even-sized slices. Spread the apple purée over the base of the tart case, then arrange the apple slices in neat, concentric circles, starting from the outside. Brush the apples with butter, then scatter over the reserved sugar and bake for another 20-25 mins until golden.

STEP 5

Mix the jam with 1 tbsp hot water from a freshly boiled kettle. When the tart has finished baking, glaze generously with the jam, then leave to cool a little. Serve warm or cold, dusted with icing sugar, if you like.

Sticky pear & ginger cake

<u>Ingredients</u>

For the cake

250g stoned dates, finely chopped

300ml milk

100g butter, plus extra for the tin

140g ginger preserve (you'll find this with the jams)

140g dark muscovado sugar

3 large ripe pears (we used Conference)

175g self-raising flour

50g pecan nuts, reserve 10 and chop the rest

1 tsp bicarbonate of soda

2 tsp ground ginger

½ tsp mixed spice

2 eggs, beaten

For the brandy syrup

85g light muscovado sugar

150ml brandy

How to Make

STEP 1

Put the chopped dates in a pan with the milk, butter, ginger preserve and dark muscovado. Heat gently until the butter has melted and the mixture starts to bubble round the edges of the pan. Stir well and set aside for 1 hr to cool.

STEP 2

Heat oven to 180C/160C fan/gas 4. Line the base of a buttered 23cm springform tin with baking parchment. Peel and chop the pears into large chunks. Mix the flour, chopped pecans and bicarb with the spices, then stir into the cooled date mixture with the eggs. Pour into the tin and scatter over the pears. Roughly break the reserved pecans and drop on top. Bake for 40 mins, then cover the top loosely with foil and return to the oven for 25-30 mins more until a skewer inserted into the centre comes out with just sticky crumbs – the cake may still look a little wet around the pears.

STEP 3

While the cake is baking, make the brandy syrup. Tip the light muscovado sugar into a pan with 50ml water and dissolve over a low heat until syrupy. Stir in the brandy and set aside. When the cake is ready, spoon over half the syrup, then leave the cake to cool before serving with extra syrup on the side.

STEP 4

To freeze, cool the cake in its tin, then wrap well and freeze for up to 3 months. Defrost and warm through in a low oven. The syrup can be frozen separately, warmed, then drizzled over as before.

PART 5: FINAL THOUGHTS

In wrapping up, facing esophagitis can be a real challenge, but you're not alone in this journey. Coping with this condition requires a blend of patience, persistence, and a proactive stance toward your well-being.

For anyone grappling with esophagitis, my heart goes out to you, and I want to offer my genuine support and encouragement. Navigating life with a digestive issue is tough, no doubt, but each day offers a chance to take positive strides toward managing symptoms and enhancing your overall quality of life.

It's crucial to team up with healthcare professionals to craft a personalized treatment roadmap that meets your unique needs and circumstances. Whether it's tweaking your diet, embracing stress-relief practices, or leaning on your support network, know that there are options available to help you better handle the ups and downs of esophagitis.

Remember to be gentle with yourself and celebrate even the smallest victories along the way. Healing isn't always a swift process, but with your determination and resilience, relief is within reach. Keep your spirits up, stay strong, and hold onto the belief that brighter days are ahead.